GINSENG

MARIAN KIM

ISBN: 1508661472

ISBN-13: 978-1508661474

CONTENTS

MARIAN KIM

1

AMERICAN GINSENG

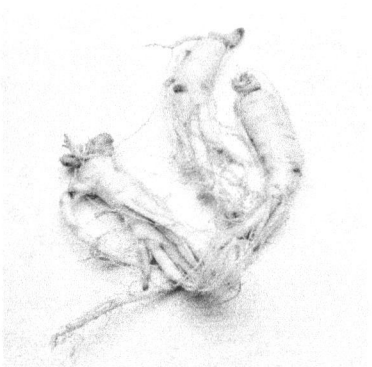

American Ginseng

American ginseng: Panax quinquefolius

Other names: Man root, anchi ginseng, ginseng root

American Ginseng Properties

Anti-aging properties

Anti-cancer properties

Analgesic (pain relieving) properties

Aphrodisiac

American Ginseng Uses

Diabetes treatment

A study found that patients with type 2 diabetes who took 3 grams of American ginseng before a meal had lower fasting blood sugar levels and lower glycosylated hemoglobin levels than those who did not.

Colds and flu prevention

American ginseng is used to prevent colds and flus. It also makes their symptoms milder and helps them last for a shorter duration if they do occur. Ginseng decoction and ginseng syrup can be prepared for this purpose.

Infection management

American ginseng is used to manage infections like HIV/AIDS, dysentery and Pseudomonas infections that commonly occur in persons with cystic fibrosis.

Anorexia treatment

American ginseng is used to improve the appetite in persons with anorexia.

Gastritis and colitis treatment

American ginseng is used for gastritis (inflammation of the stomach) and colitis (inflammation of the colon). It is also used for vomiting.

Digestive aid

American ginseng is used to improve digestion. Ginseng decoction can be prepared for this purpose.

Memory aid

American ginseng has been shown to improve short-term memory.

Menopause symptom treatment

100 mg to 500 mg of Ginseng taken three times a day has been used to manage menopausal symptoms. American ginseng combined with other herbs like black cohosh, dong quai, red clover and chasteberry tree was also found to reduce the hot flashes and night sweats of menopause.

Anti-aging aid

American ginseng is used as an anti-aging aid.

Anemia treatment

American ginseng is used for iron deficiency anemia. It is also used for bleeding disorders.

Dizziness treatment

American ginseng is used to treat dizziness.

Pain relief

American ginseng is used to treat nerve pain. It is also used for headaches, painful joints and fibromyalgia.

Erectile dysfunction treatment

American ginseng is used to treat erectile dysfunction (ED).

Fever treatment

American ginseng is used for fever.

Hangover treatment

American ginseng is used to reduce the symptoms of hangover.

Attention Deficit Hyperactivity Disorder (ADHD) treatment

American ginseng is used to treat ADHD.

Cancer treatment aid

Chinese studies showed that women with breast cancer who took American ginseng or Asian ginseng did better and felt better. Ginseng also has anti-cancer properties.

Stress management

American ginseng is used for stress management since it helps establish a sense of calmness and emotional wellbeing.

American Ginseng Safety Precautions

1. Do not use/ avoid American ginseng if you have breast cancer, cancer of the ovaries, uterus or any other hormone sensitive cancer or hormone sensitive condition like uterine fibroids and endometriosis. This is due to the fact that some American ginseng herbal preparations contain ginsenosides which act like the hormone estrogen in the body and can worsen these conditions.

2. Do not use/ avoid American ginseng if you are pregnant since one of the chemicals found in its relative the Asian ginseng has been linked to birth defects.

3. Do not use/ avoid American ginseng if you are breastfeeding since not much is known about its safety.

4. Do not use/ avoid American ginseng if you have insomnia or trouble falling asleep and staying asleep since it has been linked to insomnia.

5. Do not use/ avoid American ginseng if you have schizophrenia because high doses have been linked to agitation and sleep problems in persons with this mental disorder.

6. Do not use/ avoid American ginseng if you are using diabetes medications since it can also lower blood glucose levels.

7. Do not use/ avoid American ginseng if you are scheduled to have surgery within 2 weeks since it can interfere with blood sugar levels.

American Ginseng Drug Interactions

1. Persons taking diabetes medications should not use/avoid American ginseng since it can also lower blood glucose levels.

2. Persons taking warfarin (coumadin) should not use American ginseng since it has been reported to decrease the effectiveness of this blood thinner.

3. Persons taking monoamine oxidase inhibitors (MAOIs) antidepressants should not use/avoid American ginseng since the combination can cause anxiety, restless and insomnia.

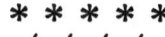

2

ASIAN GINSENG

Asian ginseng: Panax ginseng

Other names: Chinese ginseng, ginseng blanc, white ginseng

Asian Ginseng Properties

Analgesic (pain relieving) properties

Immune system boosting properties

Energy boosting properties

Anti-aging properties

Aphrodisiac

Asian Ginseng Uses

Alzheimer's disease treatment

Asian ginseng has been shown to improve mental performance win persons with Alzheimer's disease. It also improves memory in elderly persons with memory problems.

7

Improve cognitive function

Asian ginseng is used to improve concentration, abstract thinking and mental arithmetic skills. Panax ginseng improves memory when combined with ginkgo biloba. Ginseng decoction can be prepared for this purpose.

Improve athletic performance

Asian ginseng is used to improve physical stamina and athletic endurance though it does not improve exercise performance. Ginseng decoction can be prepared for this purpose.

Stress management

Asian ginseng is used for stress management since it helps establish a sense of calmness and emotional wellbeing. It is also used as a tonic for general well-being.

Depression treatment

Asian ginseng is used for depression management since it reduces feelings of sadness. It is also used for anxiety.

Chronic fatigue syndrome (CFS) treatment

Asian ginseng is used for CFS since it helps improve energy levels. It is also used for nervous exhaustion.

Cancer treatment aid

Chinese studies showed that women with breast cancer who took American ginseng or Asian ginseng did better and felt better. Ginseng also has anti-cancer properties. Panax ginseng is also thought to prevent cancers of the stomach, lung, liver, ovary and skin.

Immune booster

Asian ginseng is also known for its immune boosting effects. Korean red ginseng which is a type of Asian ginseng is thought to increase the function of the immune system in persons with HIV. Therefore, consider taking 150 -300 mg per day after consulting your doctor.

Common cold prevention

Asian ginseng extracts have been shown to reduce the risk of catching a cold. Ginseng decoction and ginseng syrup can be prepared for this purpose.

Infection management

Asian ginseng is used to manage infections like the Pseudomonas infections that commonly occur in persons with cystic fibrosis. It is also used for bronchitis.

Cancer treatment aid

Asian ginseng has been used to treat breast cancer and prevent cancers of the ovary, liver, lung and skin.

Anemia treatment

Asian ginseng has been used to treat anemia. It is also used for bleeding disorders.

Diabetes treatment

Asian ginseng has been used to treat diabetes.

Gastritis treatment

Asian ginseng has been used to treat gastritis (inflammation of the stomach lining). It is also used for vomiting.

Fever treatment

Asian ginseng has been used to treat fever.

Hangover treatment

Asian ginseng has been used to treat hangovers.

Asthma treatment

Asian ginseng has been used to treat asthma. It is also used to improve the symptoms of chronic obstructive pulmonary disease (COPD).

Anorexia treatment

Asian ginseng has been used to treat anorexia or loss of appetite.

Dizziness treatment

Asian ginseng is used to treat dizziness.

Pain relief

Asian ginseng is used to treat painful conditions like neuralgia (nerve pain), headaches, painful joints and fibromyalgia.

Menopausal symptoms relief

Asian ginseng is used to relieve symptoms of menopause like fatigue, insomnia and depression.

Anti-aging aid

Asian ginseng is used as an anti-aging aid.

Impotence treatment

Asian ginseng is used to treat erectile dysfunction (ED). It is also used for premature ejaculation. Panax ginseng also improves sexual arousal and satisfaction in postmenopausal women.

Heart failure treatment

Asian ginseng is given intravenously (in the vein) to treat heart failure.

Fluid retention treatment

Asian ginseng is used for fluid retention.

High blood pressure treatment

Asian ginseng is used to treat high blood pressure.

Halitosis treatment

Asian ginseng is used to treat halitosis or bad breath caused by Helicobacter pylori (H. pylori).

Asian Ginseng Safety Precautions

1. Do not use Asian ginseng if you are pregnant since one of its chemicals has been linked to birth defects in animals.

2. Do not use/avoid Asian ginseng if you are breastfeeding because not much is known about its safety profile.

3. Do not give Asian ginseng to children since it has caused poisoning in babies.

4. Do not use/avoid Asian ginseng if you have an autoimmune disease like systemic lupus erythematosus (SLE), multiple sclerosis or rheumatoid arthritis since it boosts the immune system and it can worsen the diseases.

5. Do not use/ avoid Asian ginseng if you have had an organ transplant since it boosts the immune system and can increase the chances of the organ being rejected.

6. Do not use/avoid Asian ginseng if you have heart rhythm problems since it can affect it on the first day of its use.

7. Do not use/avoid Asian ginseng if you have high blood pressure since it can lower blood pressure.

8. Do not use/avoid Asian ginseng if you have diabetes since it can lower blood glucose.

9. Do not use/ avoid Asian ginseng if you have breast cancer, cancer of the ovaries, uterus or any other hormone sensitive cancer or hormone sensitive condition like uterine fibroids and endometriosis. This is due to the fact it can act like the hormone estrogen and worsen these conditions.

10. Do not use/ avoid Asian ginseng if you have insomnia or trouble falling asleep and staying asleep since it has been linked to insomnia.

11. Do not use/ avoid Asian ginseng if you have schizophrenia because high doses have been linked to agitation and sleep problems in persons with this mental disorder.

12. Do not use/ avoid Asian ginseng if you have a bleeding disorder since it can interfere with the clotting of blood.

Asian Ginseng Drug Interactions

1. Persons taking insulin and other diabetes medications should avoid Asian ginseng since it can lower blood glucose levels.

2. Persons taking medications that slow blood clotting should not use Asian ginseng since it can also slow blood clotting. Examples include aspirin, heparin, clopidogrel (Plavix), diclofenac, dalteparin (Fragmin), enoxaparin (Lovenox) and warfarin (Coumadin).

3. Persons taking monoamine oxidase inhibitors (MAOIs) antidepressants should not use/avoid Asian ginseng since the combination can cause anxiety, restless and insomnia.

4. Persons taking furosemide (Lasix) should not use/avoid Asian ginseng it can decrease the effectiveness of furosemide.

5. Persons taking medications changed by the liver should avoid Asian ginseng since it can increase their effects and side effects. Examples include amitriptyline, clozapine (Clozaril), codeine, fentanyl (Duragesic), fluoxetine (Prozac) and tramadol (Ultram).

6. Persons taking immunosuppresants should avoid Asian ginseng since it can decrease their effectiveness. Examples include azathioprine (Imuran), cyclosporine (Sandimmune), mycophenolate (CellCept), tacrolimus (Prograf) and prednisone (Deltasone).

7. Persons taking stimulant s should avoid Asian ginseng since the combination causes increased heart rate and high blood pressure. Examples include epinephrine/ adrenaline and pseudoephedrine.

8. Persons taking caffeine should avoid Asian ginseng as the combination increases heart rate, irritability, high blood pressure.

9. Persons taking alcohol should not use/avoid Asian ginseng since it can increase how fast the body gets rid of alcohol.

* * * * *

3

SIBERIAN GINSENG

Siberian ginseng: Eleutherococcus senticosus

Other names: Ciwujia root, devil's bush, shigoka, touch-me-not, wild pepper

Siberian Ginseng Properties

Immune boosting properties

Sedative properties

Siberian Ginseng Uses

Herpes simplex 2 treatment

Siberian ginseng extract is used to treat the number, severity and duration of herpes simplex type 2 (HSV 2) infection.

Weight loss

Siberian ginseng is used for weight loss because it increases energy levels and boost the body's metabolism. This helps the body burn more fat even when it is resting. It is also thought to help the body adjust to a new weight loss program. Ginseng also enhances physical stamina and this helps a person exercise for longer.

Atherosclerosis treatment

Siberian ginseng is used for atherosclerosis (hardening of the arteries) treatment.

Rheumatic heart disease

Siberian ginseng is used for rheumatic heart disease.

Kidney disease

Siberian ginseng is used for kidney disease.

Alzheimer's disease

Siberian ginseng is used for Alzheimer's disease.

Attention Deficit Hyperactivity Disorder (ADHD)

Siberian ginseng is used for AHDH.

Diabetes

Siberian ginseng is used for diabetes.

Fibromyalgia

Siberian ginseng is used for fibromyalgia.

Rheumatoid arthritis

Siberian ginseng is used for rheumatoid arthritis.

Colds and flu

Siberian ginseng is used to relieve the symptoms of the common colds when used together with andrographis. It is also used to prevent colds.

Siberian ginseng is also used for chronic bronchitis and tuberculosis. Ginseng decoction and ginseng syrup can be prepared for this purpose.

Cancer treatment aide

Siberian ginseng is used to treat the side effects of chemotherapy for cancer patients.

Improve athletic performance

Siberian ginseng is used to improve athletic performance. Ginseng decoction can be prepared for this purpose.

Insomnia treatment

Siberian ginseng is used to treat insomnia (sleeplessness).

Immune system booster

Siberian ginseng is used to boost the immune system.

Anorexia treatment

Siberian ginseng is used to treat anorexia and increase the appetite.

Siberian Ginseng Safety Precautions

1. Do not use/ avoid Siberian ginseng if you have breast cancer, cancer of the ovaries, cancer of the uterus or any other hormone sensitive cancer or hormone sensitive condition like uterine fibroids and endometriosis. This is due to the fact that it can act like the hormone estrogen in the body and can worsen these conditions.

2. Do not use/ avoid Siberian ginseng if you are pregnant or breastfeeding for the simple reason that not enough is known about their safety profiles in these conditions.

3. Do not use/ avoid Siberian ginseng if you have high blood pressure since it can raise blood pressure.

4. Do not use/avoid Siberian ginseng if you have heart conditions like atherosclerosis and previous heart attacks since it can cause irregular heartbeats.

5. Do not use/ avoid Siberian ginseng if you have schizophrenia or mania since it can worsen these condition.

6. Do not use/ avoid Siberian ginseng if you have diabetes since it can affect blood sugar levels.

Siberian Ginseng Drug Interactions

1. Persons taking lithium should not use/avoid Siberian ginseng since it can reduce the excretion of lithium and thus increase its effects and side effects.

2. Persons taking insulin and other diabetes medications should not use/avoid Siberian ginseng since it can raise or lower blood glucose levels.

3. Persons taking medications that slow blood clotting should not use/avoid Siberian ginseng since it can also slow blood clotting. Examples of such medications include aspirin, heparin, clopidogrel (Plavix), diclofenac (Voltaren), dalteparin (Fragmin), enoxaparin (Lovenox) and warfarin (Coumadin).

4. Persons taking sedatives or CNS depressants like zolpidem (Ambien), phenobarbital, clonazepam (Klonopin) and lorazepam (Ativan) should not use/avoid Siberian ginseng since it can also cause sleepiness.

5. Persons taking medications changed by the liver should not use/avoid Siberian ginseng since it can increase the effects and side effects. Examples of such medications include clozapine (Clozaril), haloperidol (Haldol), imipramine (Tofranil) and propranolol (Inderal). amitriptyline (Elavil), codeine,

6. Persons taking alcohol should not use/avoid Siberian ginseng since it can increase the sleepiness caused by alcohol.

4

HERBAL RECIPES

Ginseng Tea

Equipment

Tea pot or kettle

***

Ingredients

1 teaspoon of ginseng powder or slices

1 cup of boiling water

Honey to taste (optional)

***

Instructions

1. Put the ginseng in a tea pot or kettle, add the boiling water and let it steep while covered for 5 or more minutes.

2. Strain and add honey (if using) to suit your taste before drinking.

*****

Ginseng Decoction

Equipment

Non-reactive heavy saucepan

***

Ingredients

1 oz (30 grams) Ginseng, chopped roots

2 pints (1000 ml) water

***

Instructions

1. Place the ginseng and water in the saucepan, cover them and slowly bring the mixture to a simmering boil for 20 minutes.

2. Remove from the heat source and let the mixture cool to drinking temperature.

3. Strain the mixture, measure it and pour the liquid into a clean saucepan.

4. Heat the liquid until it begins to steam. Reduce the heat and let the liquid continue to steam until it is reduced to half its original volume. This may take 45 minutes to 1 hour.

5. Pour the decoction into a clean bottle.

6. Store the decoction in the refrigerator to lengthen its life.

*****

Ginseng Syrup

Equipment

Saucepan

Jar with airtight lid

***

Ingredients

1 quart (1000 ml) filtered water

1 cup ginseng

1 cup honey

***

Instructions

1. Place the water and ginseng in a saucepan and bring to a boil.

2. Reduce the heat and let it simmer while it is partially covered until the volume is reduced to half the original volume.

3. Strain the mixture through a sieve or cheesecloth to remove the ginseng.

4. Measure 1 pint (500 mls) of the liquid and add the honey.

5. Cook for a few minutes as you stir it so that it thickens.

6. Store the syrup in an airtight container in the fridge for up to 2 months.

*****

Ginseng Tincture

Equipment

Glass jar with tight fitting lid

Dark tincture bottles

Cheesecloth

***

Ingredients

7 oz (200 gm) of dried ginseng or 14 oz (400 gm) of fresh ginseng

30 oz (1 liter) of 80-100 proof vodka

***

Instructions

1. Fill 1/3 of the glass jar with the chopped ginseng.

2. Add the vodka to completely fill the jar to the top.

3. Seal the jar and label it with the date of preparation and name of herb (ginseng) used.

4. Store the glass jar in a dark place for 6 weeks ensuring that you shake them weekly.

5. After 6 weeks strain out the ginseng with a cheesecloth and pour the tincture into dark tincture bottles.

6. Label the tincture bottles and store them away from light and heat.

*****

Ginseng Infused Oil

Equipment

Double boiler

Large glass bowl

Sieve and cheesecloth

Sterilized dark jars

***

Ingredients

16 fl oz. (500 ml) vegetable oil like organic olive, sweet almond oil or sunflower oil

16 oz. (500 grams) slightly bruised fresh ginseng

***

Instructions

1. Place the ginseng and oil in the glass bowl ensuring that the oil covers the ginseng. Simmer them in a double boiler for one hour at a temperature of around 120 degrees Fahrenheit (49 degrees Celsius). Do not let the mixture boil. You can repeat this step several times after letting the oils cool to create more concentrated herb infused oils.

2. Strain the mixture through a sieve and cheesecloth into a dark jar as you squeeze out as much oil as you can from the cloth.

3. Label your jars and store your ginseng infused oils in a cool dark place or in the refrigerator and use them within 3 months.

*****

Ginseng Salve

Equipment

Double boiler

Large glass bowl

Sterilized dark jars or tins

***

Ingredients

8 oz. (250 ml or 1 cup) ginseng infused vegetable oil (see previous recipe)

1 oz. (30 grams) beeswax

10 drops essential oils like lavender essential oil (optional natural fragrance)

***

Instructions

1. Place the beeswax and ginseng infused oil in the glass bowl and melt them in a double boiler.

2. Once melted remove from the heat source, allow to cool and add the essential oils (if using).

3. Pour the melted oils into the storage jars or tins and allow to cool completely.

4. Store the salves in a cool dark place.

###

ABOUT THE AUTHOR

Marian Kim is an experienced alternative medicine practitioner.

*****

OTHER BOOKS BY THE AUTHOR

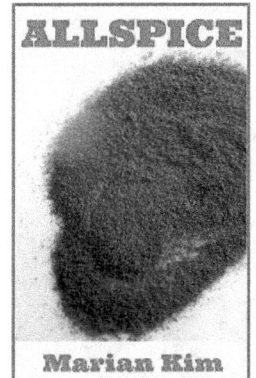
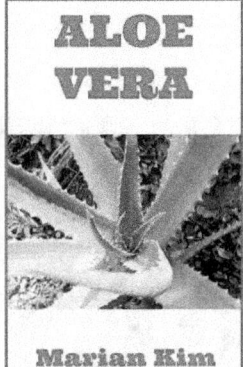
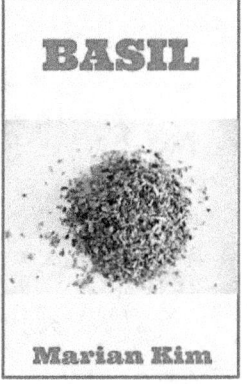

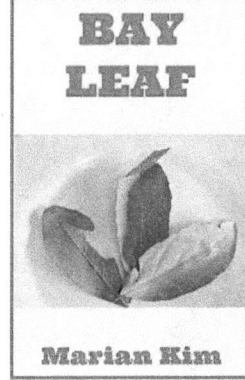
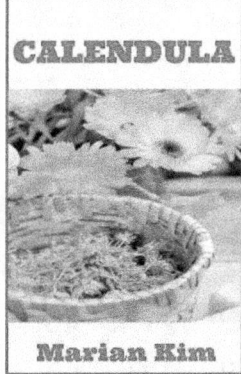
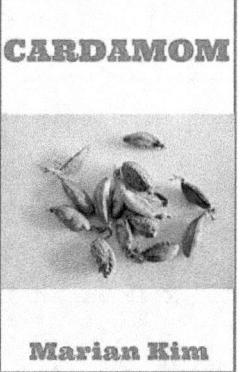

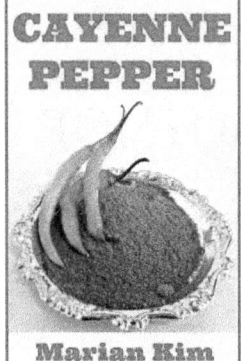

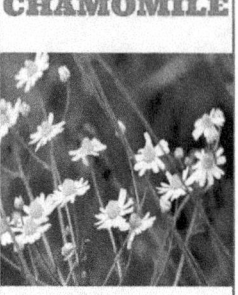

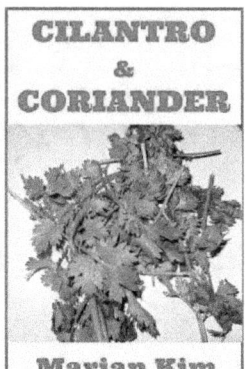

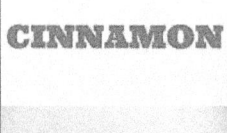

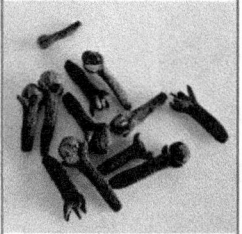

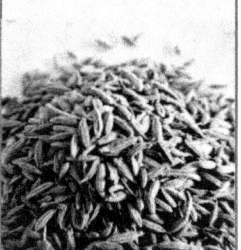

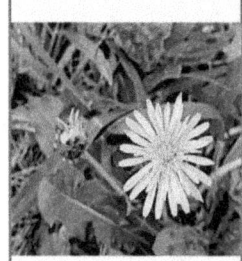

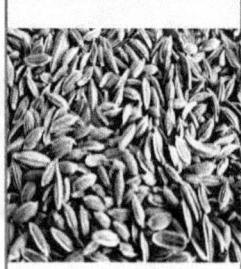

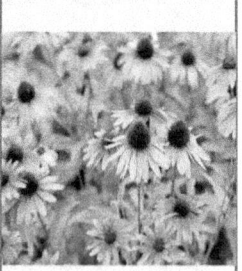

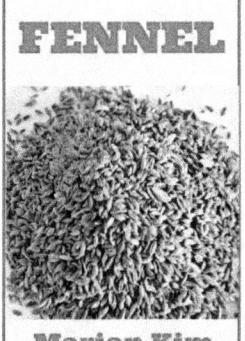

FENNEL

Marian Kim

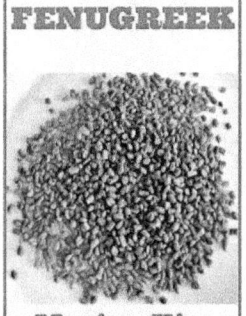

FENUGREEK

Marian Kim

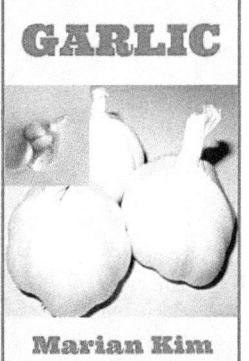

GARLIC

Marian Kim

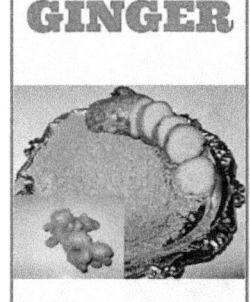

GINGER

Marian Kim

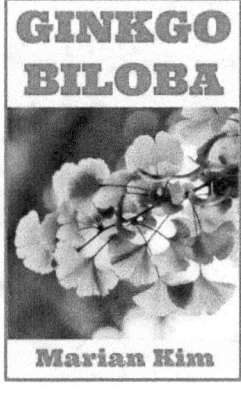

GINKGO BILOBA

Marian Kim

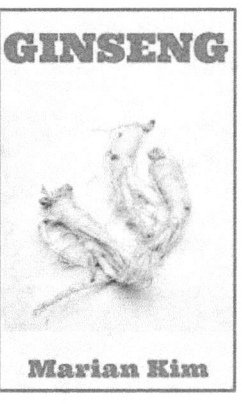

GINSENG

Marian Kim

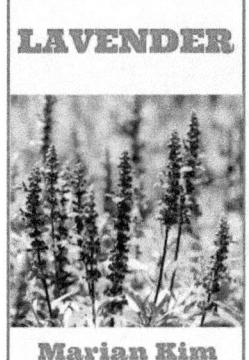

LAVENDER

Marian Kim

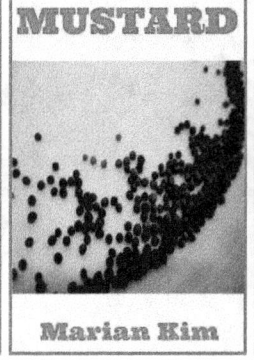

MUSTARD

Marian Kim

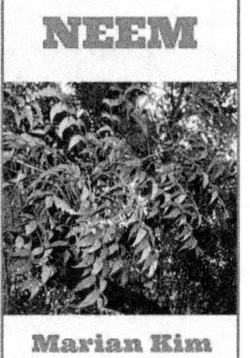

NEEM

Marian Kim

NUTMEG & MACE

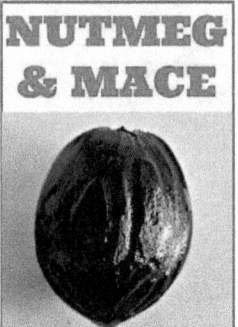

Marian Kim

OREGANO

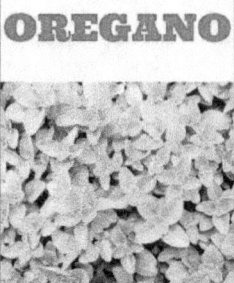

Marian Kim

PAPRIKA

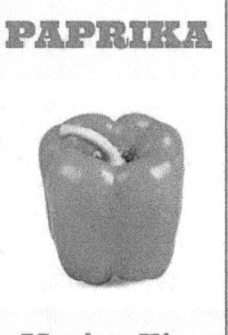

Marian Kim

PARSLEY

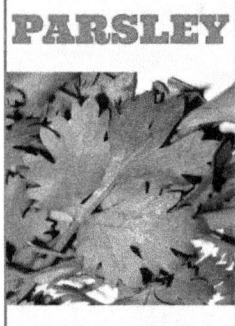

Marian Kim

BLACK & WHITE PEPPER

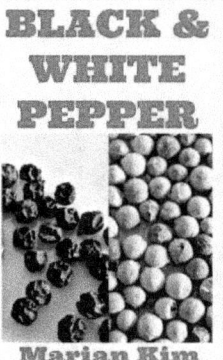

Marian Kim

PEPPERMINT

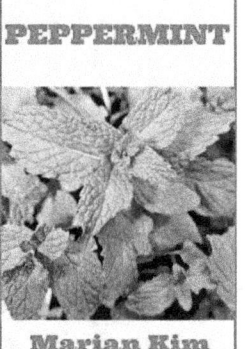

Marian Kim

ROSE HIPS

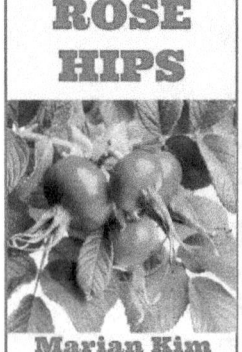

Marian Kim

ROSE PETALS

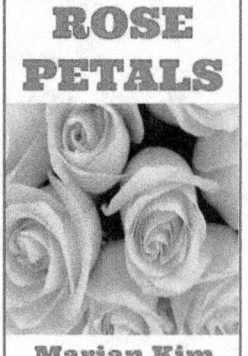

Marian Kim

ROSEMARY

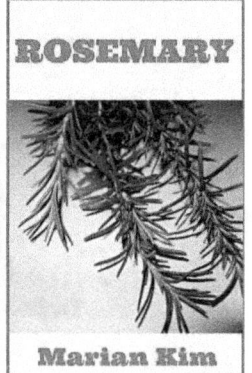

Marian Kim

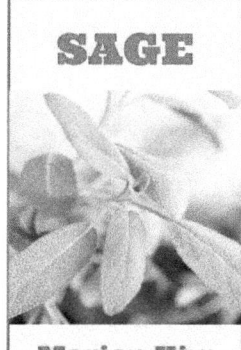

SAGE

Marian Kim

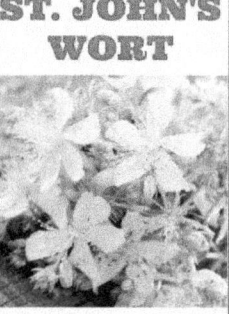

ST. JOHN'S WORT

Marian Kim

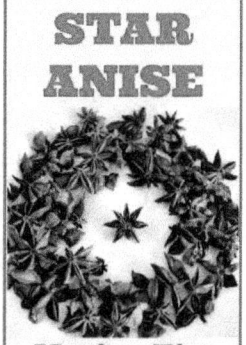

STAR ANISE

Marian Kim

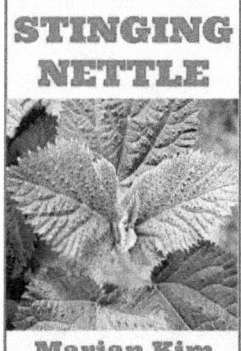

STINGING NETTLE

Marian Kim

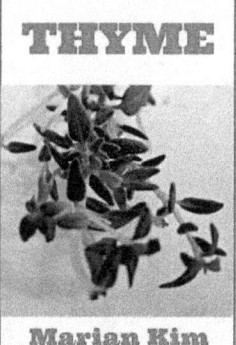

THYME

Marian Kim

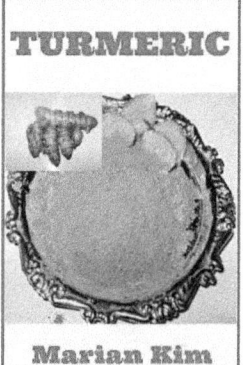

TURMERIC

Marian Kim

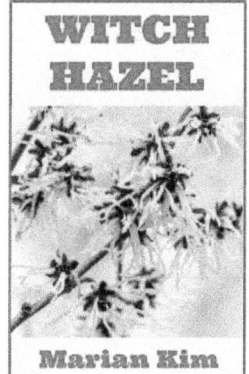

WITCH HAZEL

Marian Kim

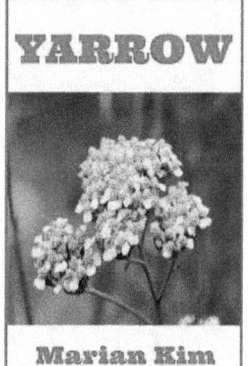

YARROW

Marian Kim

*****

www.ingramcontent.com/pod-product-compliance
Lightning Source LLC
Chambersburg PA
CBHW070516290526
45790CB00003B/1240